Full Body Massage for Beginners: The Ea
Relieve Tensions" is the ultimate guide for anyone looking to learn
the fundamentals of giving a deeply enjoyable therapeutic massage.

Written by **licensed masseur therapist Arthur Yosh**, this book is
filled with easy-to-follow instructions and beautiful illustrations of
each **massage technique**, making it the perfect guide for beginners.

With this guide, you'll be able to relieve pain, reduce tension, incre-
se relaxation, and recover and prepare for physical activities.

You'll also learn how to create a relaxing environment and connect
with your loved ones through the healing power of massage therapy.

Whether you want to give a massage to yourself, your partner, or a
friend, this book empowers you to take charge of your own health
nd well-being.

t's the perfect tool for anyone looking to reduce stress, promote
elaxation, and experience the many benefits of massage therapy.

o why wait?

tart your journey to relaxation and self-care today with
Whole Body Massage for Beginners „.

Introduction

Stress, the fast pace of life, and negative daily experiences have a destructive effect not only on the psyche but also on the body and the general efficiency of the organism.

An appropriate message - in this case a relaxation one - helps our body fight the effects of **stress and muscle tension excellently.**

Peace in the form of massage should soothe the nervous system, prepare for rest and peaceful sleep, and calm and release the muscular system and the whole body from excessive tension.

Relaxation massage

Relaxation massage includes specialist massage techniques or a specific method in which we positively influence the physical condition of the person being massaged and indirectly their emotional state through direct, gentle massage.

During the massage for relaxation, additional elements such as **aromatherapy** and **music therapy** are used. Candle, aroma, scent, incense, fragrant oils, warm bedding are not only the current fashion for relaxation, but also a condition for the massage to take place at all.

In therapeutic practice, we encounter situations where relaxation massage is used as a prelude to other cosmetic treatments, and also (lately more and more often) is used in aesthetic medicine.

Relaxation allows for a more complete diagnosis of both the condition of tissues and the whole organism, also affects acceptance and love of one's own body as it is.

Relaxation Massage Of The Whole Body

Relaxation massage should act on different levels:

Physical - functional reduction of muscle tension, soft tissues, and pain therapy.

Emotional - whole body relaxation combined with calming thoughts, relaxation and calming and revitalization.

Mental - more complete feeling of one's own body, and deepening of awareness and psychosomatic reactions, anti-stress action.

Before starting the massage, it is important to know:

- ✓ Check if the person being massaged has any contraindications to massage.
- ✓ Do not massage directly after a meal.
- ✓ Ensure the comfort and convenience of the person being massaged.
- ✓ Adapt the touch and pressure to the body and sensations of the person being massaged.
- ✓ Remember to massage in the direction of the heart or the nearest lymph nodes.
- ✓ Monitor the time of the massage, focusing on each part of the body - **the total massage time should not be less than 45 minutes (preparation and massage)**.
- ✓ Interfuse caressing with other techniques and cover the massaged part of the body so it does not cool down.
- ✓ Position the body so as to achieve maximum relaxation.
- ✓ The movements should be slow, smooth, soft, and elastic, and the touch warm and pleasant.

Relaxation Massage Of The Whole Body

Contraindications to massage:

- Weakness or exhaustion after a viral infection.
- Fever.
- Skin infections, such as itching, herpes, psoriasis.
- Inflammatory, purulent, and allergic skin conditions and all dermatological changes.
- Malignant and benign tumors.
- Cardio-respiratory insufficiency and heart defects.
- Advanced atherosclerosis of peripheral vessels.
- Hemophilia.
- Thrombosis of veins, arteries, and fresh thrombus.
- Lymph node inflammation.
- Women in their first trimester of pregnancy.
- After surgical procedures.
- In conditions threatening to bleed.
- During menstruation.
- Fresh trauma - fractures, dislocations.
- Acute cases of sciatica.
- Advanced discopathy.

CAUTION!

Massage should not be done after a **heavy meal** or after **drinking alcohol**, nor immediately **after exercise**.

This will avoid unpleasant sensations and adverse effects that may occur.

Indications

Relaxation massage is done to achieve a state of **relaxation.** The basic assumption of massage is to restore the organism's homestatic balance.

Through this type of massage, we influence the equalization of blood pressure, improvement of lymph flow, calming of the autonomic nervous system, and leveling of the hormonal system.

It is very often done in states of nervous excitability, all kinds of neuroses, excessive stress, and nervous tension, and in cases of subjective feeling of psychophysical fatigue.

Relaxation massages offer many possibilities - they can serve as preventive, diagnostic, and preparatory massages for other treatments.

Conditions conducive to relaxation during the massage

The temperature of the room.

The temperature of the place where the massage will be done is very important, as a too-cold room can cause the muscles of the person being massaged to not relax fully and for them to be cold.

The room should be well-**ventilated** and **warm.**

We can preheat towels to cover the body - this will contribute to relaxation and maximum relaxation of the whole body.

The temperature should be around 22°C.

Lighting

Ordinary daily lighting can be too harsh and can interrupt rest, a the same time tiring the eyes.

The lighting must be adapted to the time of day - late in the evening, dimmed light is recommended, such as a nightlight or scattered scented candles, which will add atmosphere.

Peace and quiet

Some people will prefer subdued, relaxing background **music**, others complete peace and silence to be able to relax and unwind

The most important thing is that nothing distracts or annoys the person being massaged.

Necessary equipment and accessories

- towels
- cosmetic oil, cream or massage gel - sliding agents
- blanket or warm coverlet to cover the body
- a roller, pillow or folded towel to place under the knees in lying on the back or under the feet in lying on the stomach
- aromatherapy set, essential oils, scented candles

POSITIONING POSITIONS FOR MASSAGE

ying on the stomach: the arms are arranged in a position that is omfortable for the person being massaged - along the torso, on ne side, or in front.

roller or folded towel is placed under the feet to relax the legs. the bed does not have a hole in the face, the head should be laced sideways towards the masseur.

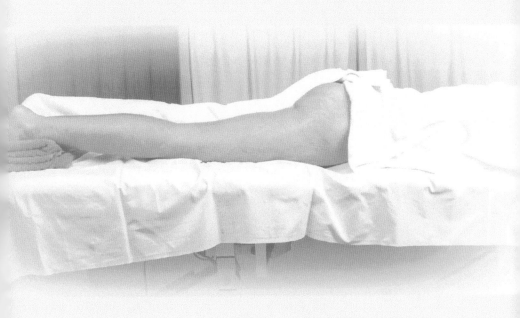

this position, we massage the **calf, back of the thigh, but-cks, and back along with the neck.**

POSITIONING POSITIONS FOR MASSAGE

Lying on your back: the head is supported on a slightly raised headboard, and the arms are held along the torso.

A **roller or folded towel** is placed under the knees to relax the legs.

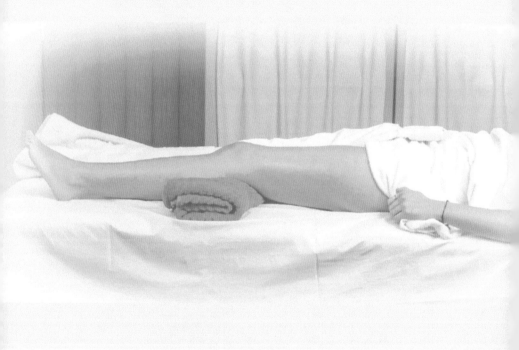

In this position, we massage the **dorsal side of the foot, the front of the thigh, the thigh, the abdomen, and the chest, as well as the arms.**

Techniques of Relaxation Massage

Techniques of Relaxation Massage

IMPORTANT!
**remember that the massage should be pleasant and relaxing,
 must not cause pain or muscle tension. The hand movements
 hould be slow and precise.**

STROKE

his technique is always used to start and end the massage.

. With both hands, stroke longitudinally along the massaged
 ea.
. With both hands, stroke transversely to the side, perpendicu-
 rly to the massaged area.

ules of Stroking

stroking can be gentle (superficial) and energetic (deep),
 epending on the force of the pressure.

stroking is used to start the massage in order to warm up
 e body and get used to the masseur's hand.

stroking should be interspersed with other techniques and
 ould end the massage gently.

this technique is performed without pressure.

the masseur's hands should be arranged freely and loosely
 ingers connected, the whole hand resting on the body).

Techniques of Relaxation Massage

In a relaxation massage, various forms of stroking are often used, interspersed with other techniques, which act more strongly and deeply on tissues.

Stroking should maintain the body in a state of relaxation and rest while maintaining the heat of the massaged part of the body.

FRICTION

This is a technique of deep and precise massage, always used after stroking and before kneading.

1. Circular with the thumb - circular movements, clockwise, moving slowly along or across the massaged area.

2. Circular with fingertips - circular outward movements made with both hands simultaneously or alternately, moving slowly along or across the massaged area.

Rules of Friction

- it is a technique of circular-push movements.
- causes the formation of a skin fold in which stretching and rubbing of the massaged tissue occurs.
- its direction is determined on the basis of the anatomical structure of the massaged (muscles, joints).
- the friction rate is about 60-100 strokes per minute.
- tight contact with the massaged tissue is important, no slipping is allowed.

KNEADING

hese are movements of lifting, pressing, and squeezing the
assaged tissue

Wave kneading with both hands - with one hand, grab the
kin, with the fingers of the other hand hold the skin fold - then
nange hands.

Simultaneous kneading with both hands - with both hands
multaneously grab the skin, then lift it and then lower it.

Pinch kneading with both hands - simultaneously with the
umbs and index fingers grab the skin fold, then release and
lax.

les of Kneading

- it is most often used to massage muscles.
- it is important that the massaging hand softly grab the
ssues and lift and squeeze them without pain.
- the masseur's hands should move smoothly, without slip-
ng, across the massaged area.
- tempo 40-50 strokes per minute.

SHAKING AND VIBRATIONS

Causing trembling of tissues by elastic shaking of the massaged area.

1. Labile vibration - with one hand support, cause vibrations w the other, moving the fingertips across or along the muscle, without lifting the hand from the massaged body.

2. Shaking - with spread and loosely arranged fingers, shake th massaged body (with one hand or both hands along the massag muscle or to the side).

3. Squeezing - with one or both hands squeeze and squeeze th tissues, moving along or across the massaged muscle, without losing contact with the skin.

Rules of Shaking and Vibrations.

 these are vibrations of small amplitude.

 require a lot of effort from the masseur.

METHODOLOGY OF RELAXATION MASSAGE

CTION PLAN

Lower limb - back of the right and left leg.

Spine - whole back.

Lower limb - front of the right and left leg.

Abdomen.

Chest.

Upper limb - right and left arm.

me of the whole massage - from 45 to 60 minutes (prepara-
on and massage)

Lower limb - back

Lying on the stomach.

1. Long stroking - we start from the heel and move our hands along the leg to the buttocks, avoiding the knee joint.

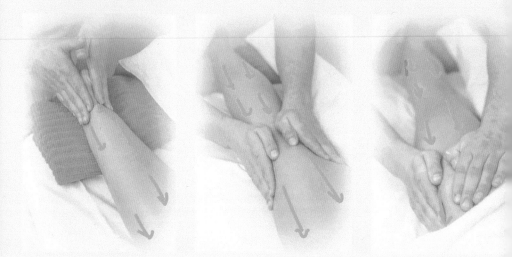

2. Cross stroking - we stand on the side of the table, on the farther side, perpendicular to the leg. We make a movement from the heel sideways (from one side to the other), moving to the thigh and then to the buttocks. Cross stroking can be done with both hands simultaneously or alternately.

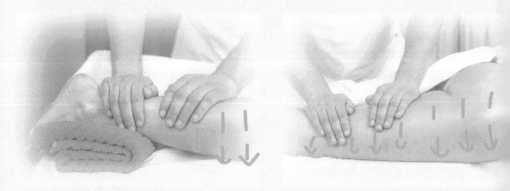

Circular kneading with thumbs - we start from the heel, along the leg (avoiding the knee joint), to the buttocks. Circular movements can be done with thumbs simultaneously or alternately.

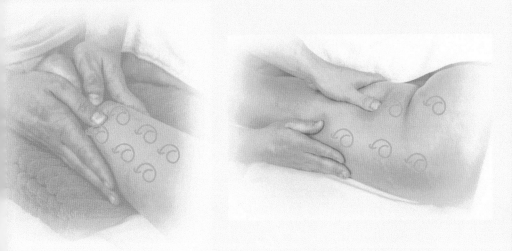

Circular kneading with fingertips - we start from the heel, along the leg (avoiding the knee joint), through the back of the thigh to the buttocks. We make circular movements with fingertips simultaneously or alternately.

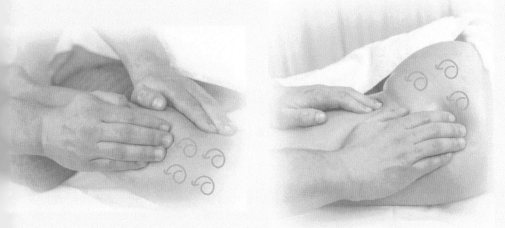

5. Double squeezing - we stand on the side of the table, on the farther side. We slide the skin fold, starting from the heel, towards the buttocks (avoiding the knee joint). We squeeze with thumbs and index fingers - the grip can be simultaneous or alternating.

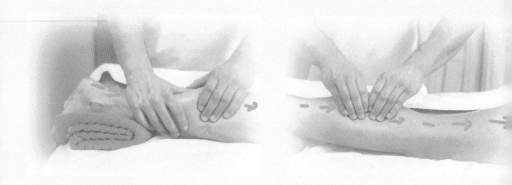

6. Shaking - with freely arranged and spaced fingers, we shake the massaged leg - we start from the heel, through the calf, thigh towards the buttocks.

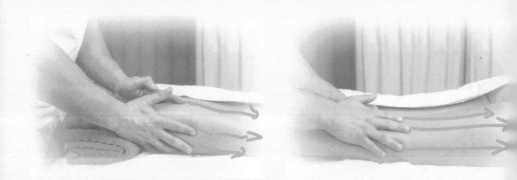

Labile vibration - we hold one hand with the other and cause vibrations. We move the fingertips along the leg, from the heel to the buttocks (avoiding the knee joint).

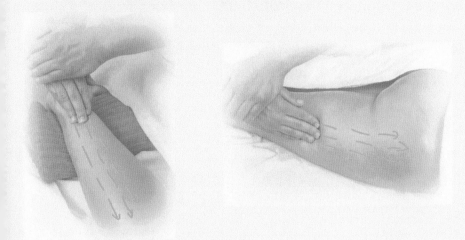

Squeezing - we put our hands in a fist; with the middle part of the fingers we lightly press the skin, moving our hands along the leg, from the heel to the buttocks (avoiding the knee joint). We maintain pressure all the time.

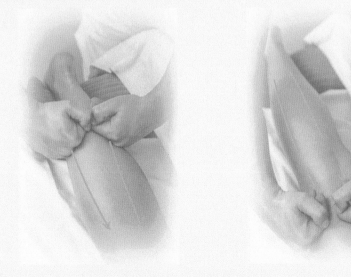

Spine

Lying on the stomach

1. Long stroking of the whole back - we start from the sacrum (lower part of the back), along the spine to the neck and occiput, descending to the shoulders. We keep one hand on one side of the back, the other on the other side.

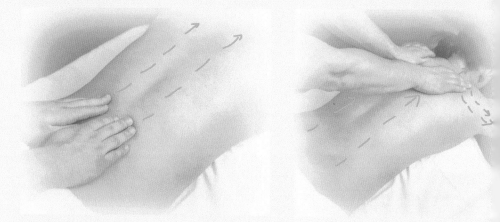

2. Cross stroking of the back - we make movements from one side to the other, dividing the back into strips. First we massage the lower part of the back (lumbar-sacral part), then the chest part and finally the upper part, i.e. cervical.

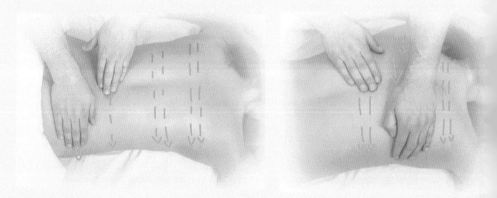

3. Cross kneading - with fingertips or thumbs we make circular or spiral movements along the hip plate, to the side of the back.

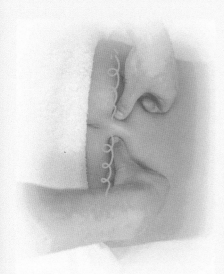
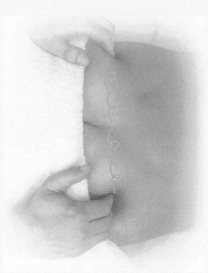

4. Long kneading - with thumbs or fingertips we make simultaneous and alternating circular movements along the spine (moving towards the head) on both sides.
Then we massage the next strip, moving away from the spine.

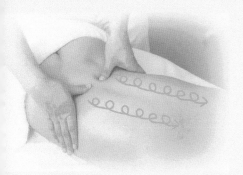
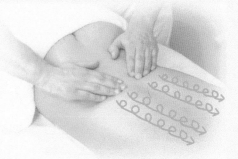

5. Circular kneading - with thumbs or fingertips we make simultaneous and alternating circular movements. We move along the neck to the occiput and to the side of the shoulders.

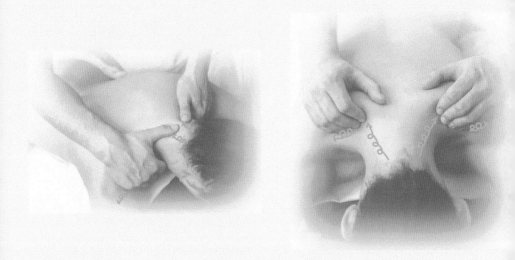

6. Wave squeezing with both hands - with the thumb of one hand we grab the skin fold, holding it with the fingers of the other hand. Then we change hands. We move along the spine or to the side.

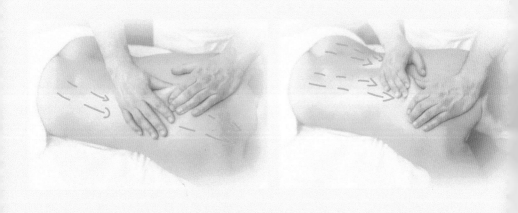

7. Wave squeezing with both hands - with the thumb of one hand we grab the skin fold, holding it with the fingers of the other hand. We move from the neck (neck) to the shoulders. Then we change hands.

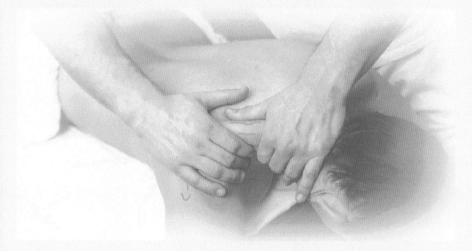

8. Labile vibration - we hold one hand with the other, which causes vibrations, moving the fingertips across or along the spine. We do not lift our hand from the massaged body.

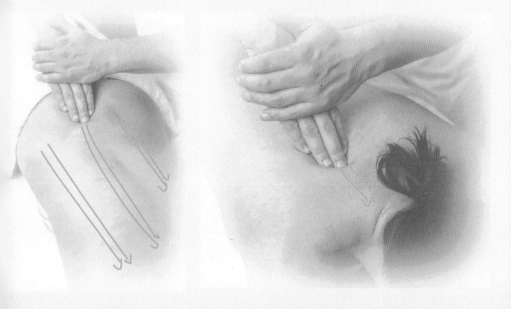

9. Shaking - with spread, freely arranged fingers, we shake the massaged body. Movements are made with one hand or both hands, along the spine or to the side.

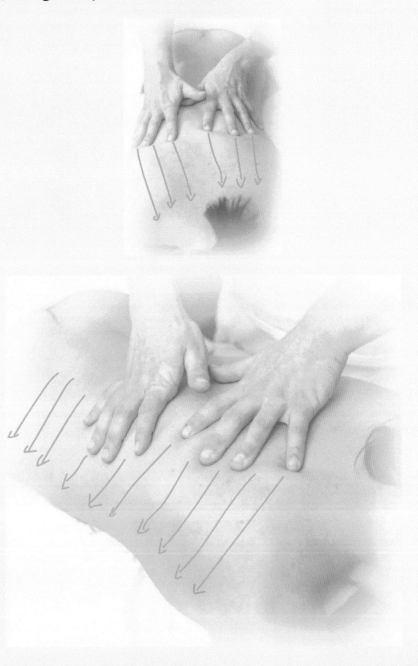

Lower limb – front

Lying on the back

1. Stroking longitudinal – we start from the dorsal side of the foot and move our hands along the leg, through the thigh to the hip.

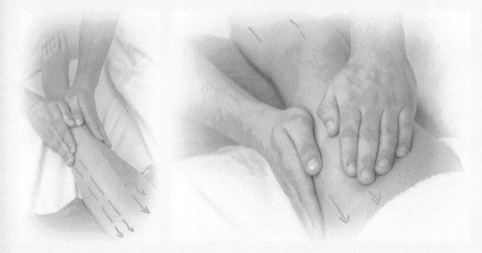

2. Cross-stroking alternate – we stand at the side of the table, on the further side, perpendicular to the leg. The movement is from the side of the foot outward, moving towards the knee, then the thigh and hip.

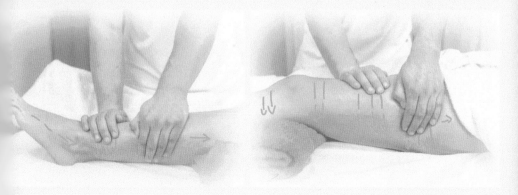

3. Kneading circular – with thumbs and fingertips perform alternate or simultaneous circular movements. We move from the dorsal side of the foot towards the thigh and hip.

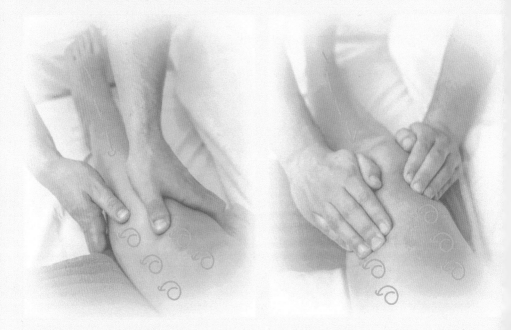

4. Wave-squeezing alternate – move the fold of skin along the leg, starting from the foot, towards the thigh and ending at the hip.

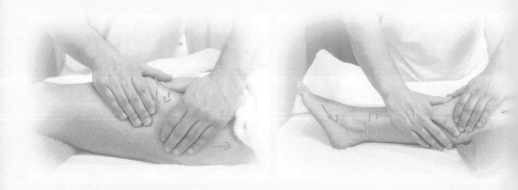

5. Labile vibration – with one hand supporting the other, we cause vibrations, moving from the toes to the hip. We do not remove the hand from the massaged body.

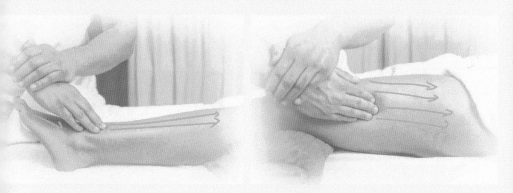

6. Shaking and squeezing – with freely spread hands we shake the skin, moving along the leg, from the foot to the hip. When squeezing, maintain pressure on the massaged body and move towards the hip.

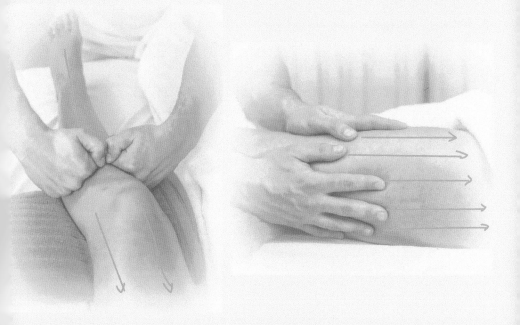

Stomach

Lying on the back

1. Cross-kneading alternate — we stand at the side of the table; massage the stomach, drawing circles. Perform movements in accordance with the clockwise.

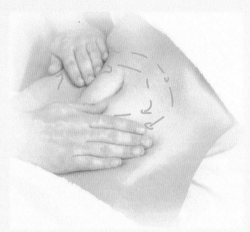

2. Kneading with one hand fingertips — one hand is held freely, with the other we perform circular movements, starting from the navel. Move outward, away from the navel.

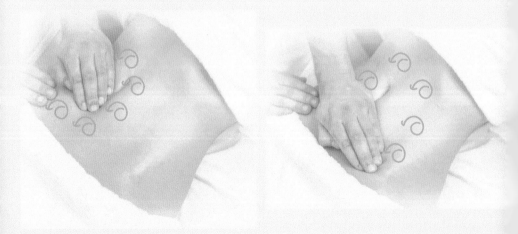

. Cross-squeezing alternate – crosswise: moving the fold of kin from the closer side to the further; longitudinal: from the ottom of the stomach to the top (towards the chest), in strips.

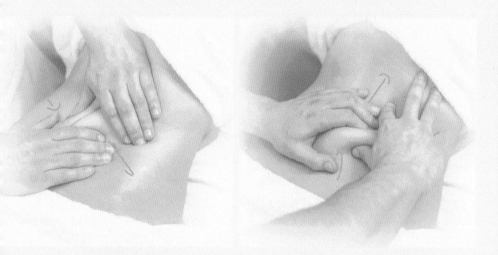

. Shaking – with freely spread fingers shake the stomach crosswise and longitudinally).
ote! When massaging the stomach, pain and too much ressure must not be caused.

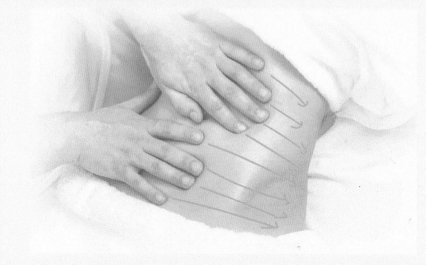

Chest

Lying on the back

1. Double stroking simultaneously – we stand behind the head; with the inner side of the hand we perform a sliding movement, moving from the middle of the chest, along the collarbone, to the shoulders.

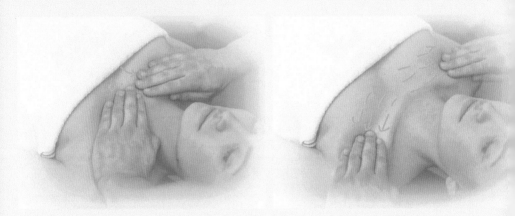

2. Double stroking simultaneously – we stand behind the head; with the outer side of the hand we perform a sliding movement, moving from the middle of the chest, along the collarbone, to the shoulders.

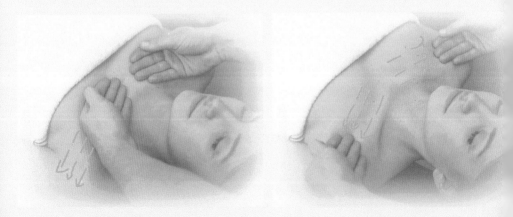

3. Circular kneading with fingertips or thumbs – perform circular movements, moving from the middle of the chest outward, along the collarbone, to the shoulders.

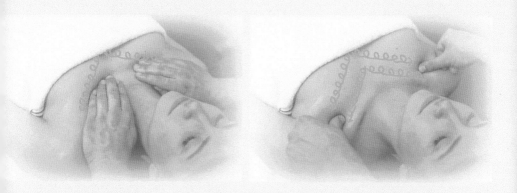

4. Labile vibration – with one hand supporting the other, causing vibrations. We move from the closer shoulder to the opposite. We avoid the collarbone.

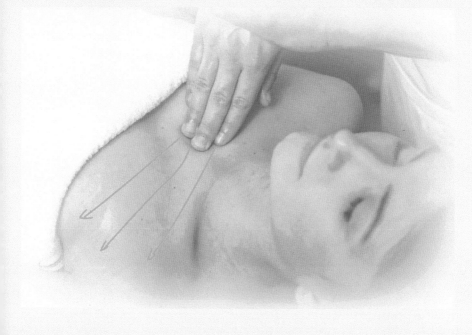

Upper limb

Lying on the back

1. Double stroking longitudinal – we start from the outer side of the hand, through the forearm, arm, to the shoulder.

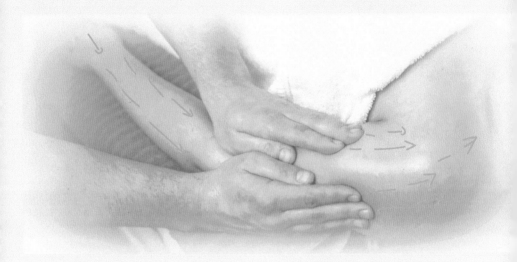

2. Double stroking crosswise – the movements are performed sideways, depending on where we stand, from the hand to the shoulder.

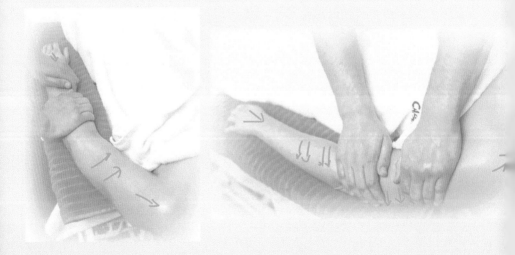

3. Circular kneading with fingertips or thumbs – perform simultaneous or alternate circular movements. We start from the outer side of the hand towards the shoulder.

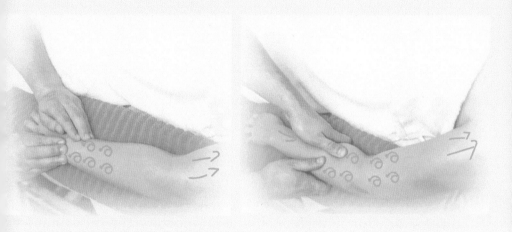

4. Wave-squeezing double-handed – we grab the skin, holding the fold of skin. We start from the hand, move towards the elbow and then to the shoulder.

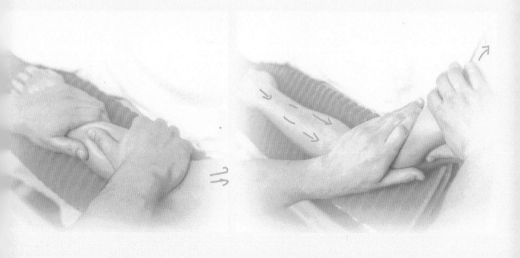

5. Double-handed pinching-squeezing simultaneously – with the thumbs and index fingers we grab the fold of skin. We move towards the elbow and then to the shoulder.

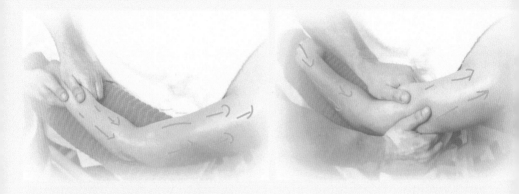

6. Labile vibration – with one hand supporting the other, causing vibrations. With fingertips we move from the hand, through the arm, to the shoulder.

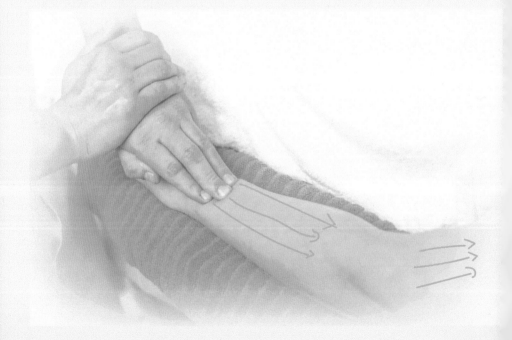

7. Shaking – with freely spread fingers gently shake the massaged part of the body. We move from the wrist, through the forearm, arm, to the shoulder.

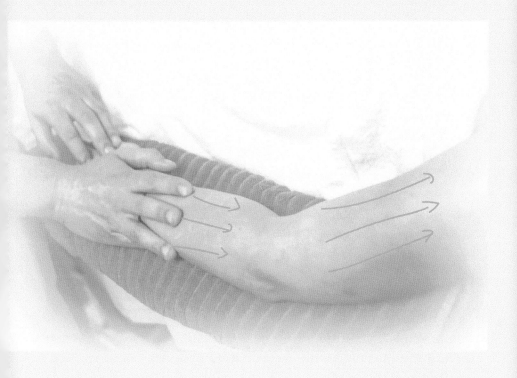

Inspirations in relaxation massages

Masaż Pantai Luar - performed on a heated bed. We use four so-called stamps, for which natural materials such as cotton and linen are used for production. Rice, coconut flakes, and spices are wrapped, and then the stamps are heated. We massage them with warm symbols, increasing the pressure as they cool down.

Masaż Lomi Lomi Nui - literally means "touch of a soft paw of a satisfied cat". Lomi techniques involve not only the hands of the masseur but also the wrists and forearms. All massage techniques are performed by the masseur in a dance-like, swaying motion. This is meant to bring the massaged person into a trance and harmony.

Thai massage - combines elements of yoga, meditation, reflexology and dietetics. Massage is done through stroking, rubbing, squeezing, stretching and lifting the relaxed parts of the body by the masseur.

Chinese cupping massage - vacuum massage with the use of cups. Due to the creation of a vacuum between the cup and the skin of the massaged person, we get the effect of congestion, and by removing the air from the cup, we improve the elasticity and firmness of the skin. The cups are usually made of rubber, due to the possibility and ease of moving them over the skin.

Tibetan bowl massage - massage based on the effects of sound. The bowls are a combination of ritual and everyday use vessels. During the massage with the bowls or other tools, the sound is emitted, which transmits sound and vibration waves to the massaged body. The vibration and soothing sound put the body into deep relaxation and oblivion.

Bamboo massage - a relaxing massage performed with sticks and brushes made of bamboo, which are rolled over the body. With posts that fit the shape of the muscles during the massage, the body is tapped, stroked, and kneaded with varying rhythm and intensity. This massage has a stimulating, relaxing, and mood-improving effect, making the body feel amazing lightness. In addition, the familiar sound of bamboo sticks puts the body into deep relaxation and forgetfulness.

Printed in Great Britain
by Amazon

40974310R00021